Sedona Reflexology Foot Massage Manual

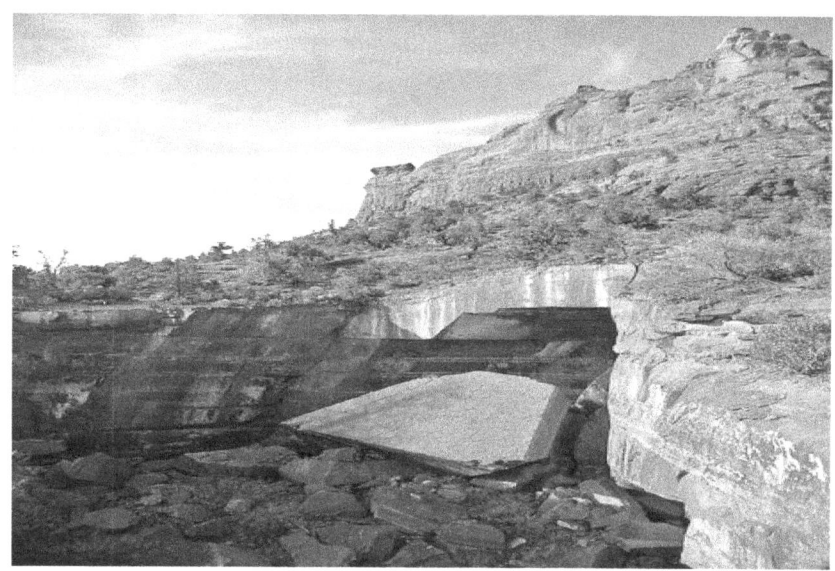

A Healing Arts Workbook For Beginners

By: Shiatsu Tom

Co- Author Reiki Marie

Original Classic Edition With Illustrations

For The Healing Arts Schools & Couples

ISBN-13: 978-1475273748
ISBN: 10:1475273746

DEDICATION

FOOT MASSAGE

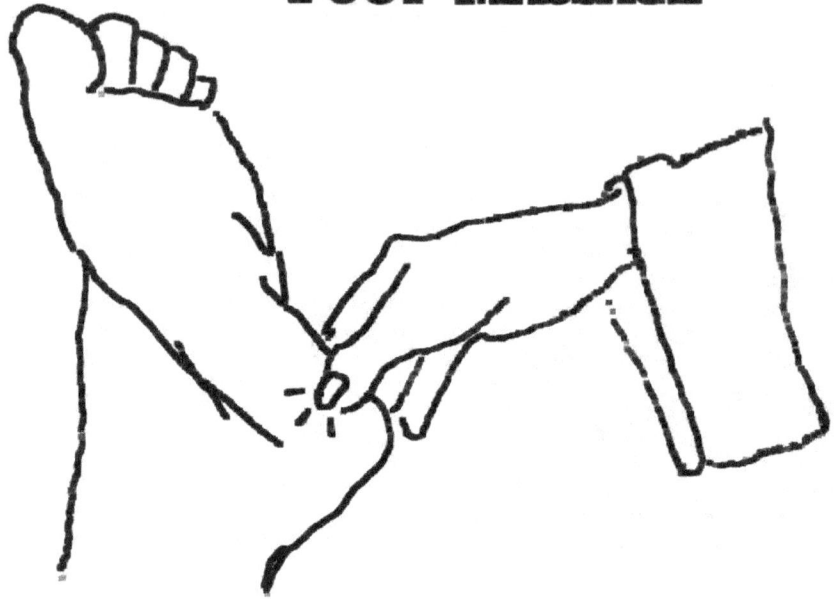

This book was written in loving memory of my son: Thomas Matthew It is designed so that you can work on yourself, or preferably on a friend, husband or wife.

With Love

Shiatsu Tom

Reiki Marie

CONTENTS

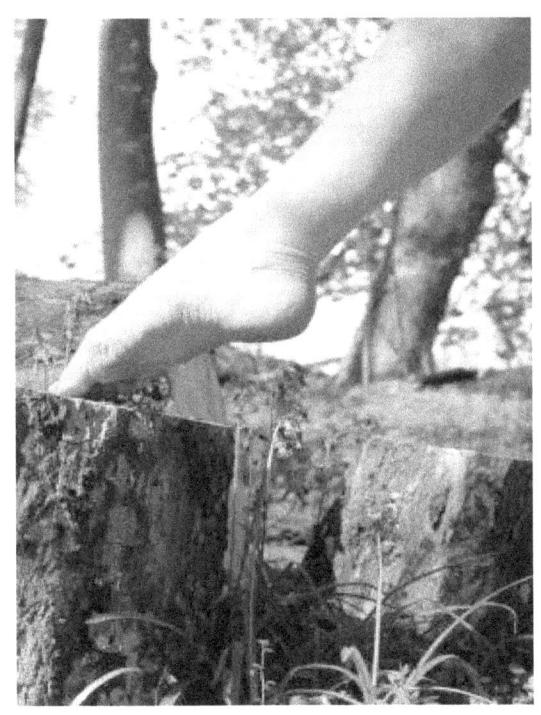

REFLEXOLOGY FOR COUPLES
OR
HEALING ART THERAPISTS

〔FOOT MASSAGE〕

INTRODUCTION

Reflexology, or zone therapy, is an alternative healing art involving the physical act of applying pressure to the feet, with specific thumb, finger, and hand techniques without the use of oil or lotion. It is based on what reflexologists claim to be a system of zones and reflex areas that they say reflect an image of the body on the feet and hands, with the premise that such work effects a physical change to the body. There is no consensus among reflexologists on how reflexology is supposed to work; a unifying theme is the idea that areas on the foot correspond to areas of the body, and that by manipulating these one can improve health through one's Qi.

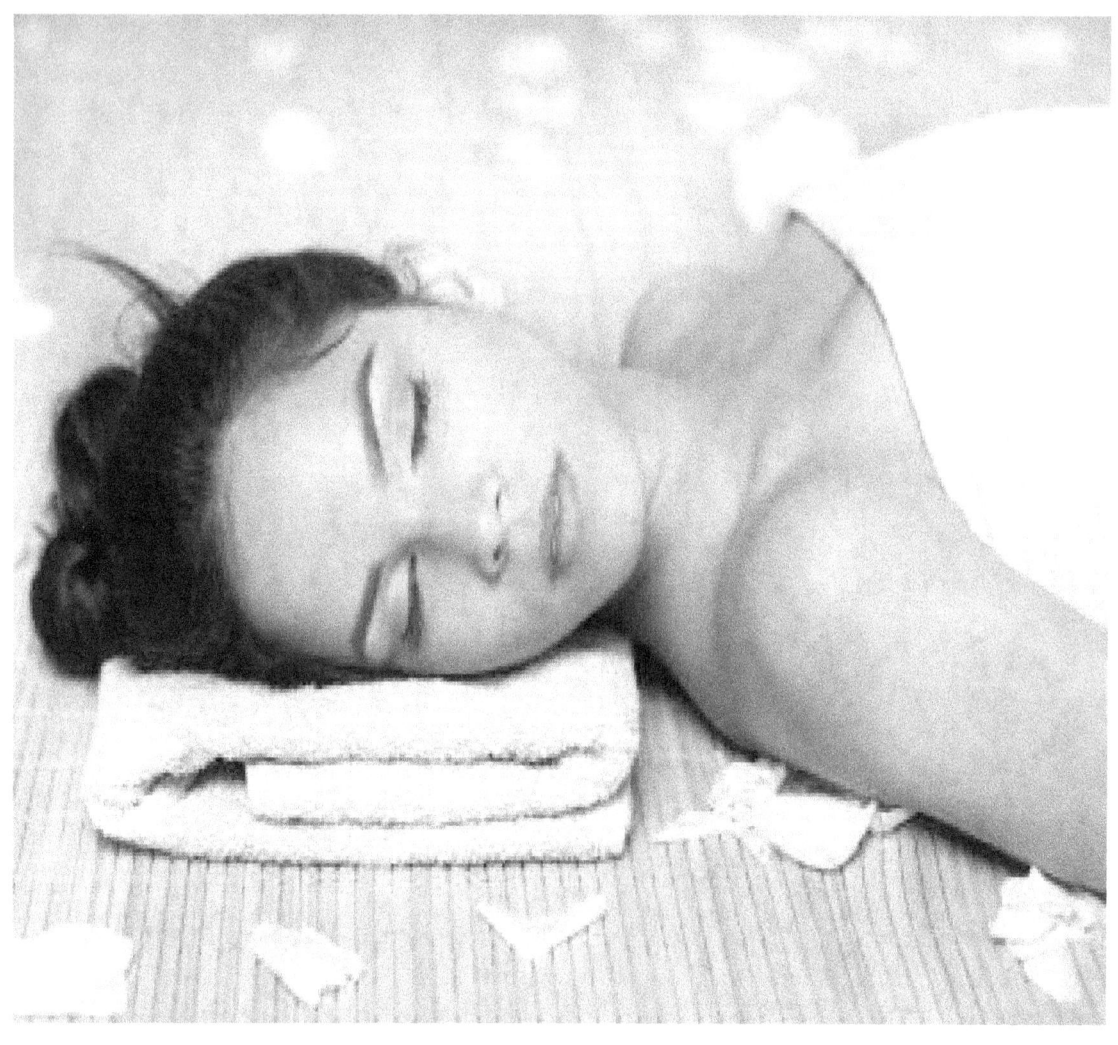

**A Simple Workbook For Learning The Art Of Reflexology.
Always Take Your Time And Practice. Remember It Can Take More Than One Reflexology Treatment To Achieve Maximum Results.**

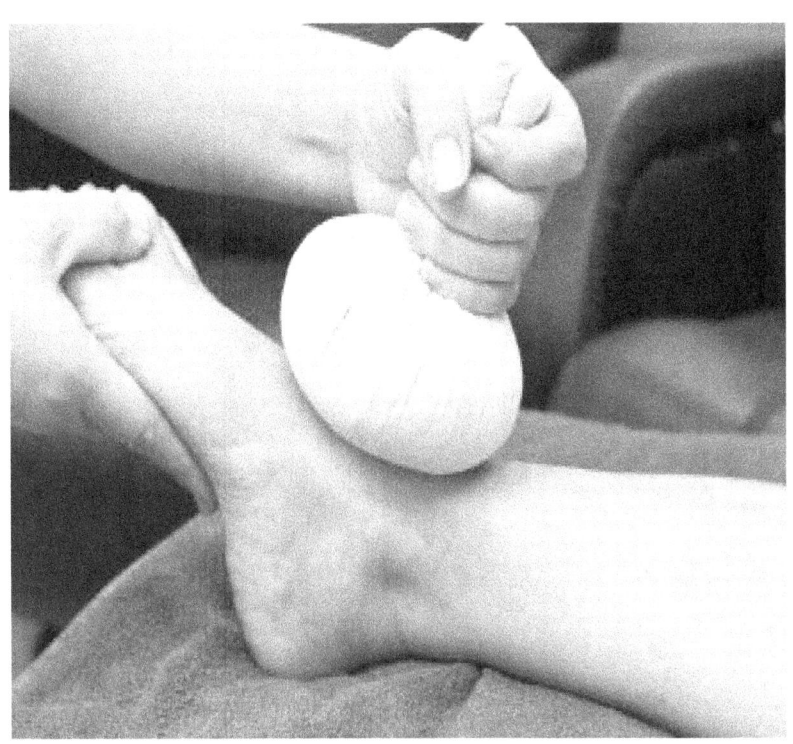

HOW DOES REFLEXOLOGY HELP?

Nerve connecting pathways to all parts of the body closest to the surface are located in the feet. These are called pressure points. Various grips permit us to reach and treat tender spots in the feet, that relaxes and normalizes functions and stimulates circulation in the feet and through-out the body. Your body's alarm system works for you. Pain, nausea, dizziness, etc...

Sometimes when these symptoms appear it is quite late because many conditions of poor health take time to develop.

Pressure points will help discover many potential physical problems in their early stages or almost before they occur.

(Important) In cases of serious or prolonged symptoms consult your doctor. Please do not try to act like a doctor. There is only one way to become a M.D. go to school. Just do your routines and you will be richly rewarded with the knowledge that you are helping others. There is no exact location for anything in our body, because some peoples feet are bigger or smaller, so we work the approximate location. Once you find one or several tender points treat the area.

If this is a boyfriend, girlfriend, husband, wife, or just a friend make it a habit to check pressure points for each other once a week, almost before they occur. Awareness of a problem in time often facilitates fast improvement.

Always take note of the locations of the tender spots. You can write them on a piece of paper (remember them). At first the checkout routine may take 30 minutes or longer. Once you become more knowledgeable of the points it takes less time. Routine maintenance helps to increase stimulation of the organs and increases circulation. Bottom line, it also increases relaxation.

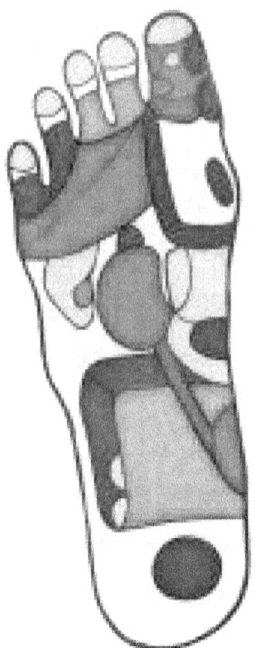
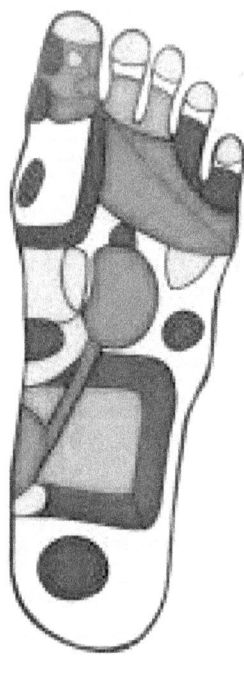

Legal Disclaimer:

This publication contains the opinions and ideas of its authors. It is intended to provide helpful and informative material on the subjects addressed in the publication. It is sold with the understanding that the authors and publisher are not engaged in rendering medical health, or any other kind of personal professional services in this book The reader should consult his or her medical, health, or other competent professional before adopting any of the suggestions in this book or drawing inferences from it. The authors and publisher specifically disclaim all responsibility for any liability, loss or risk, personal or otherwise, which is incurred as a consequence , directly or indirectly of the use and application of any of the contents of this book.

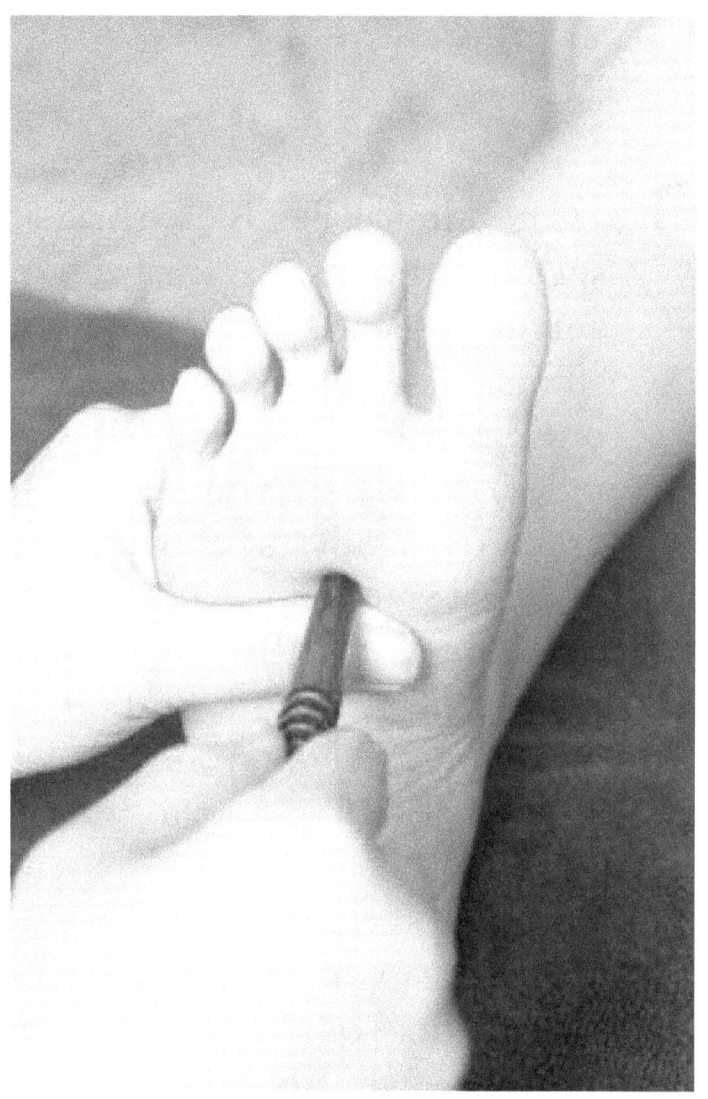

HOW DO I DO REFLEXOLOGY?

Helpful Tips and Tools

1. First it is good to cut real long finger-nails, if you wish.
2. Follow a check-out routine starting at the toes, and working to the heel.
3. Press firmly enough for the pressure to be felt. Don't cause pain with your own pressure by using too much strength. Be firm, but gentle
4. Learn how much pressure each person likes, with practice.
5. Allow plenty of time to cover the entire foot. Imagine lines from top to bottom, and across the entire foot.
6. You can use oil or lotion if you prefer to allow the thumbs to move more easily.

Tools are sometimes used. Cut a pencil to a 3 inch cut may be used. Then cut off 2/3 of the eraser, and use the eraser. Or a wooden stick as shown in the photograph. Use it on the bottom of the feet if you wish but not necessary.

SECTION 1 TECHINIQUES
ADRENAL GLANDS REFLEX=AG

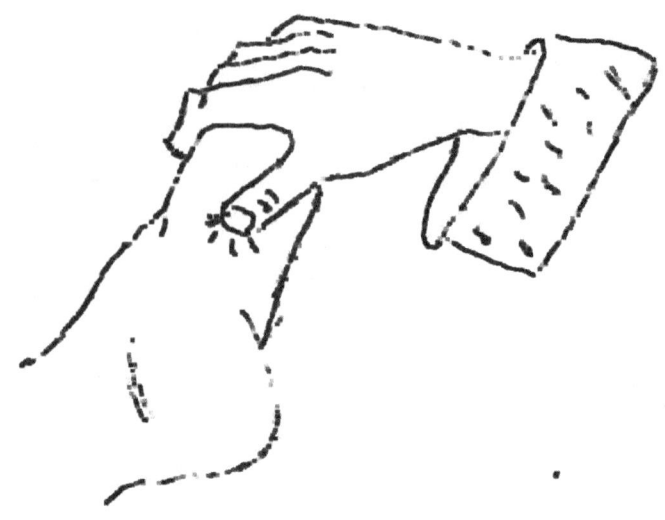

The adrenal glands are small and specific points. Visualize the adrenal gland that you are stimulating and regulate your breathing. Inhale as you press this reflex, exhale as you release the pressure. Work the point slowly and deliberately so as not to cause any real pain. Pain is often already there. Since there are two adrenal glands it is best to work on both the left and right foot. To find the adrenal point: first fix your toes and notice how a tendon forms a ridge from the ball of the foot to the heel. Move your thumb along this tendon, to a point just above ½ way between the toes and the heel in the arch of the foot. If you are working the right foot move your thumb a little to the right of the tendon. If you're on the left foot the point will be just left of the tendon. Press firmly on this point with your thumb. Press slowly and gently the first time. Release the pressure slightly, but not altogether. Just be sure to work until the soreness lets up or the soreness is gone. This will take a few practice days.

SECTION 2 TECHINIQUES
ARMS AND SHOULDERS= AS

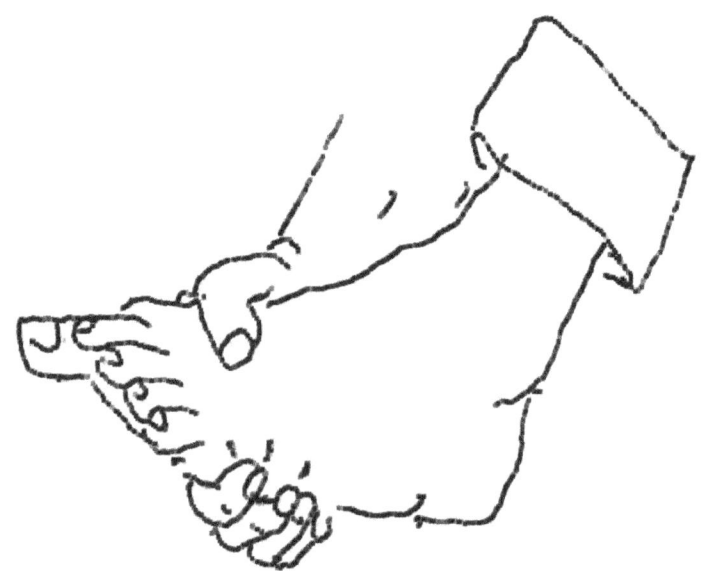

The reflex on the right foot corresponds to the right arm and shoulder. The left is for the left arm and shoulders. You should work both sides, not just one side. This will help to balance the body. Be aware of any pain or tenderness in these areas.

Work the area slowly using deliberate pressure without causing any real pain. Visualize the part of the body that you are working on. Inhale as you press the reflex area then exhaling as you release the pressure. Use your thumb to work the area. Start beneath the crease between the 4th toe and the little toe. Extend down to just below the ball of the foot at the base of the little toe. The reflex area goes all the way to the outer edge of the foot. Use your thumbs on the sole for better leverage. Press with a gentle but firm motion. Let up on the pressure just a little then press again. Do not let up on the pressure completely until the soreness lets up or it is gone.(Continue to practice often

SECTION 3 TECHNIQUES
BLADDER-URETHRA= BUU

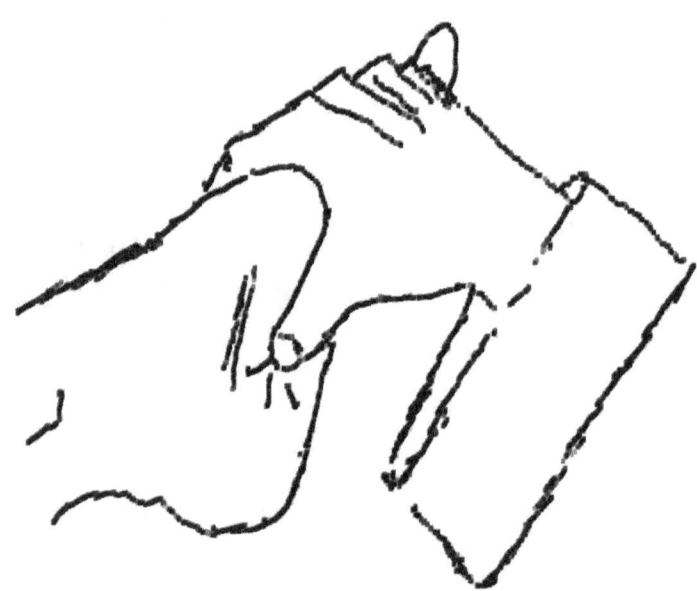

There is a strong interrelationship with the uterus, bladder and the urethra. It is best to stimulate the reflex area of all three in the same session. You will find the reflex areas on the soles of both feet. Work on both feet using your thumbs because the bladder and urethra are in the center of the body. The reflex areas are actually split between both sides of the body. The reflex point for the uterus is in the middle of the soft hollow in the arch straight down from the second toe. For the bladder and urethra, reflex is at the lower end of the arch on the edge of the foot, next to the pad of the heel. Massage the area using your thumbs with a firm but gentle pressure. Massage the area extending from the beginning of the uterus reflex over to the bladder-urethra reflex. Do this gently until soreness or discomfort is gone.

SECTION 4 TECHINIQUES
THE BRAIN REFLEX= B

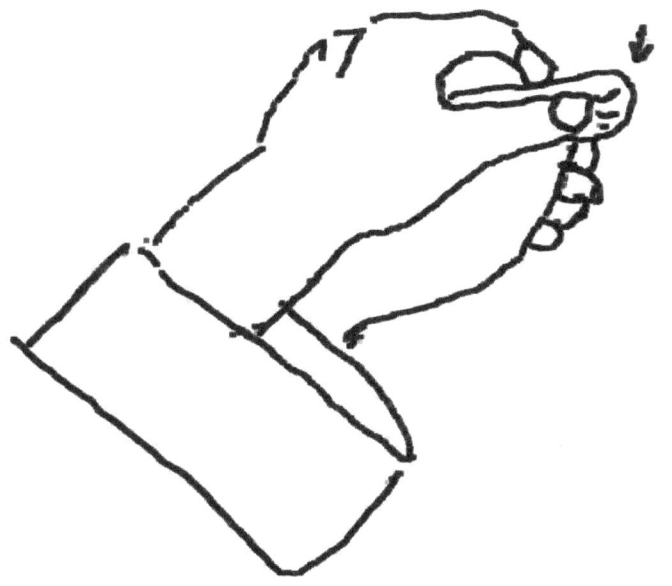

To stimulate the left side of the brain work the reflexes of the left foot. Work the reflexes of the right foot for the right side of the brain. The right side of the brain controls such intellectual functions as special orientation and creativity. The left controls analytical abilities and speech. The brain has a cross-over effect on the body. The right half affects the functions of the left side of the body. The left half- affects the functions of the right side of the body. The same as before, control your breathing. Inhale as you press the reflex and exhale as you release pressure. On both feet the brain reflex area is the large portion of the big toe. Grasp it between your thumb and with your index finger squeeze as you move to cover the entire area of the big toe. Gently but firmly. Do not release the pressure until it is relaxed. (Note: this is a very sensitive area so take your time).

SECTION 5 TECHNIQUES
THE BREAST REFLEX= BR

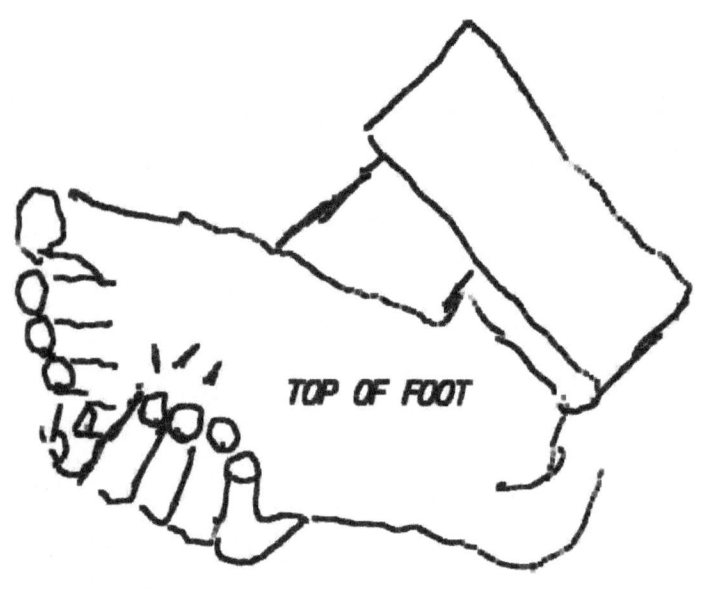

TOP OF FOOT

The breast reflex areas are located on the top of each foot. Work the areas carefully as they are extremely sensitive to pressure (rubbing is better). Take your time and be sure not to bruise the top of the foot. Control your pressure as well as your breathing. Inhale as you press the reflex and exhale as you release pressure. The breast reflex extends from the second toe across the top of the foot to about half way to the ankle. You will work the entire area. Use the palm of your hand against the sole of the foot for resistance. Use your thumb in a gentle circular motion. Control your pressure and be sure to carefully include the tendons between the bone of the foot. Rub the area of the tendons with the index finger gently and be sure to do both feet.

SECTION 6 TECHNIQUES
THE EAR REFLEX= E

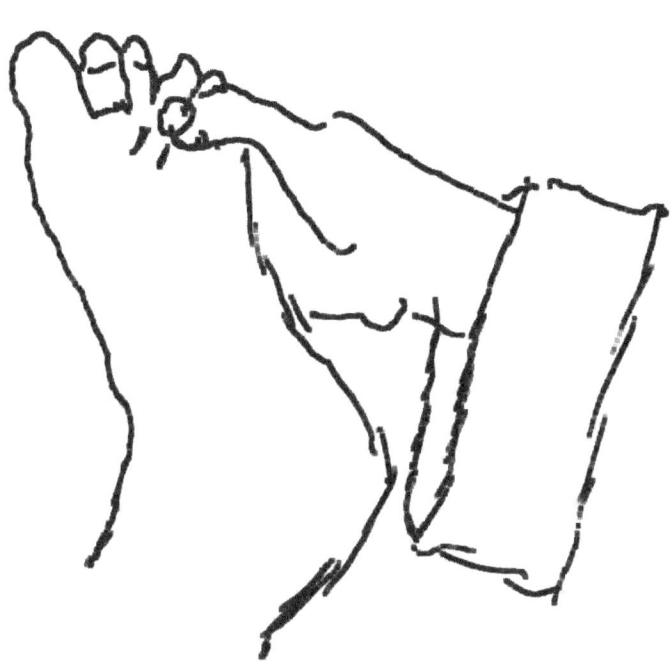

The ear reflex on the feet is a small area rather than a specific point. Work the area slowly and deliberately and take your time. Be careful not to cause any real pain and be sure to work both feet. The ear reflexes on both feet are on the soles at the base of the fourth toe. All the way over to the little toe. This also includes the rubbing between them. Place your thumb on the sole of your foot, starting at the 4th toe. Apply pressure until you reach the little toe. (squeeze, let-up, squeeze and let-up) Use your index finger to work on the rubbing between the toes gently.

SECTION 7 TECHNIQUES
THE EYE REFLEX= EY

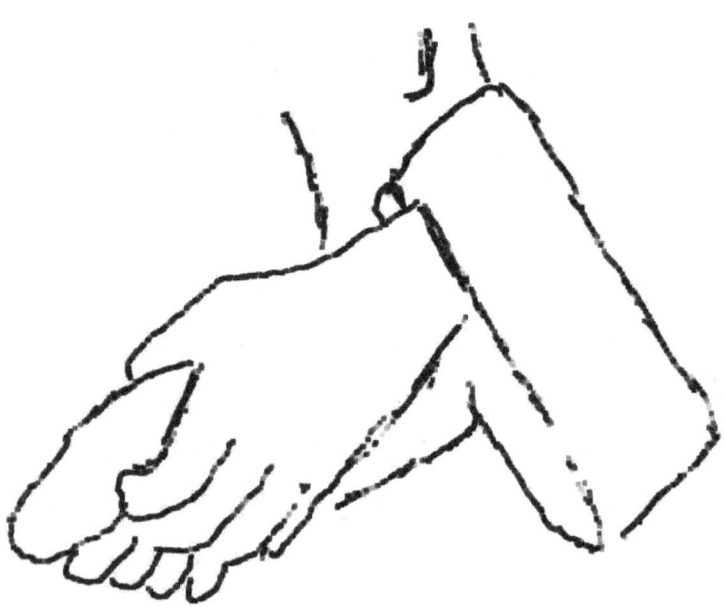

Because there are two eyes work both feet. The reflex area on the left foot stimulates the left eye. The ones on the right foot are for the right eye. (Be sure to work both feet). The eye reflex on both feet is a small area rather than a specific point. Control your breathing. Breathe in as you press the reflex and breathe out as you release the pressure. The eye reflex areas are on the right and left soles of the feet at the base of the second and third toes, include rubbing between them. Place your fingertips on the sole of your foot and use the other hand or your thumb on the opposite side to provide resistance. Exert a firm squeeze with your fingers moving back and forth over the entire reflex area. Then release pressure slightly but not altogether. Repeat several times.

SECTION 8 TECHNIQUES
GALLBLADDER REFLEX= GB

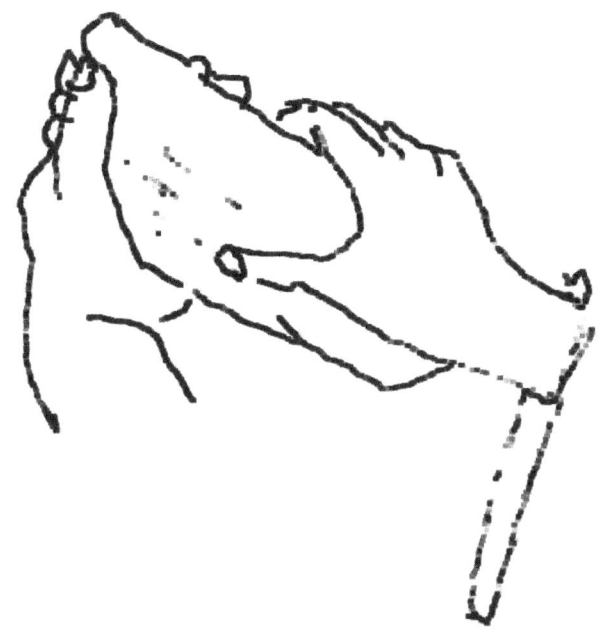

The gallbladder is a small specific point. Work the point slowly and deliberately. Be careful not to cause any real pain. To find the gallbladder point: Gently slide your thumb down the sole of your right foot. Start at the crease between your 4th toe and little toe. Stop when you are a little less than half the distance between your toes and the back of your heel. This is the gallbladder point. Use your thumb press firmly on this point. Press slowly and gently then release pressure slightly. Work until the soreness is gone. It is good to work both feet.

SECTION 9 TECHNIQUES
THE HEART REFLEX= H

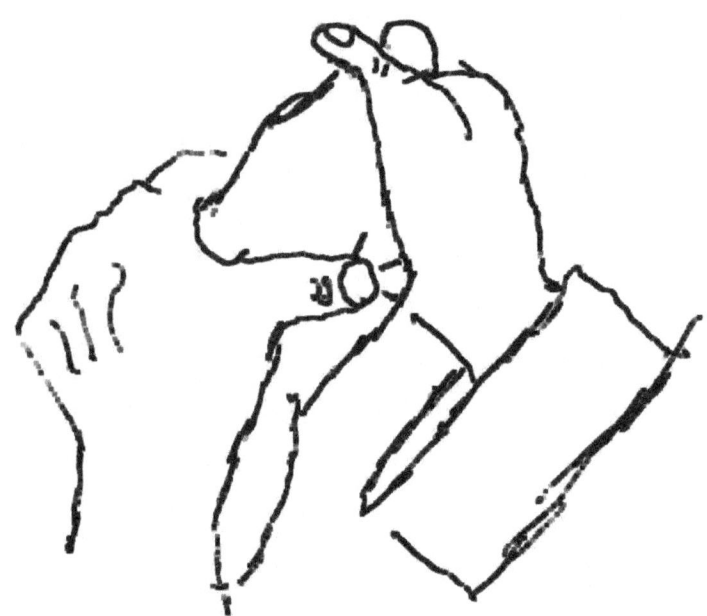

Since most of the heart is primarily on the left side of the body, the reflex point is on the left sole. Concentration on the reflex itself will yield the most direct results. Visualize the heart and its functions while stimulating the reflex. Concentrate on your breathing pattern. You will find the heart point on the sole of your left foot. Using your right hand to flex the toes place your left thumb just below the ball of the foot straight down from the (4th) toe. Use your thumb in a circular motion. Press gently and firmly on the reflex several times until the pain subsides. (Note this is a tender area so take your time and practice). It is good to work both feet.

SECTION 10 TECHNIQUES
HIPS-THIGHS-LEGS REFLEX= HTL

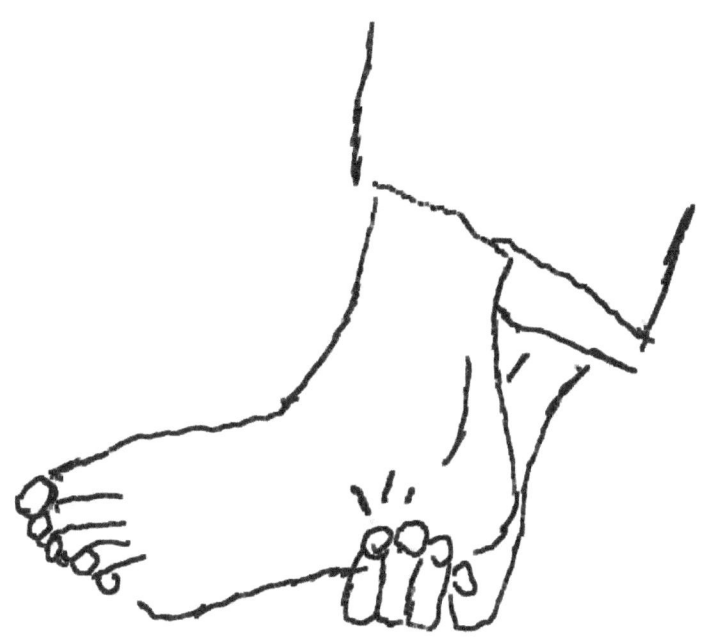

Stimulating the reflexes for the hips, thighs, and legs is a great way to invigorate them. The reflex on the right foot correspond to the right. The reflex on the left foot correspond to the left side. It is good to work both sides for each hip, thigh and legs. The reflex area for the hips, thigh, and legs can be found on the outer edge of each foot, about 1/3 of the way between the heel and the base of the toes. Extending from the sole up to about (1/2) the distance to the base of the ankle bone. Use your index, middle and ring fingers in a circular motion. Apply a firm pressure on the area and cover the entire area .Apply firm but gentle pressure. Do both feet for the best results.

SECTION 11 TECHNIQUES
INTESTINE REFLEX= IN

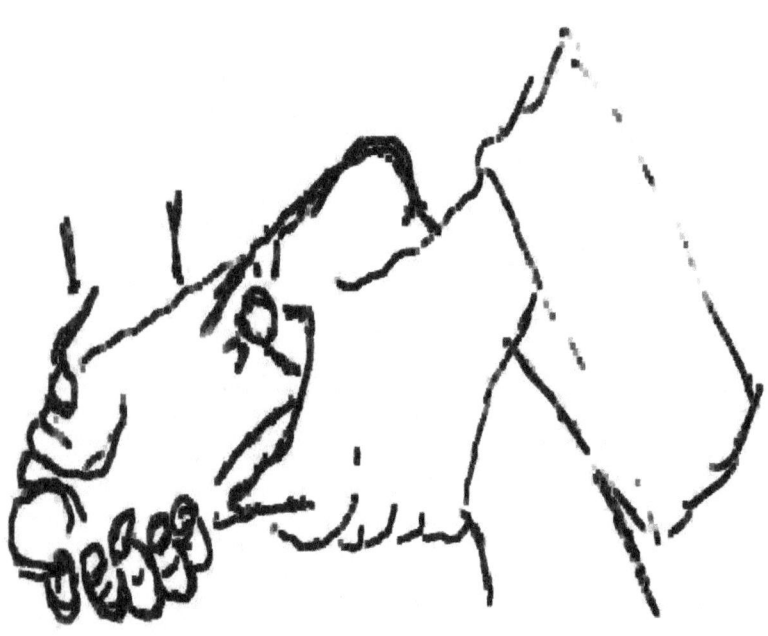

Working the intestine reflex areas: Be sure to work both sides of the body. Pay attention to the ileocaecal reflex. The ileocaecal valve opens and closes when food moves from upper to lower intestine and sometimes sticks causing great pain. Work your way around the reflex area. In a clockwise circular motion starting from the middle work both soles the intestine reflex starts near the top of the heel pad. This extends up a little more than halfway to the toes and from the inner to the outer edges of the foot. Exert firm pressure with your thumbs. Start in the center of the area and work to the outside edge.

SECTION 12 TECHNIQUES
KIDNEY REFLEX= K

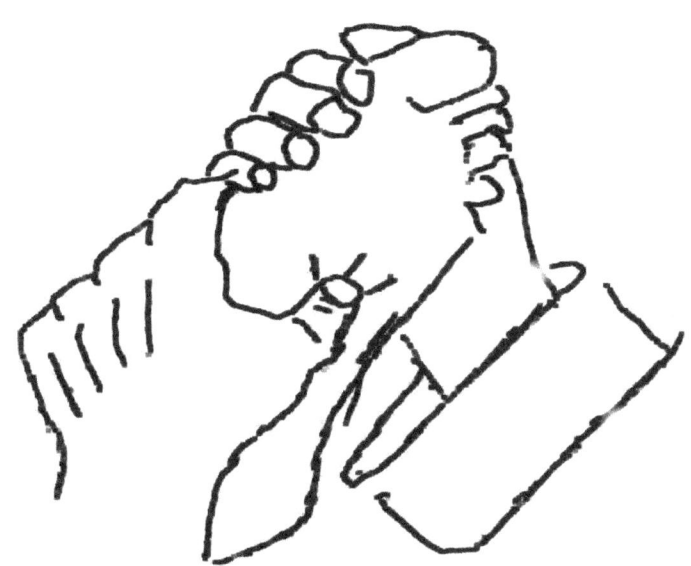

Since there are two kidney's there are reflex areas on both feet. For the most direct results concentrate on the reflex area. To find the kidney areas on both feet use one of your hands to flex the toes. You will see a tendon form a ridge. From the ball of your foot to the heel slowly move your thumb along the tendon to a soft spongy area ½ way between the ball and the heel, in the middle of the arch. This is the kidney reflex. Now un-flex your toes and the arch. Use that hand to hold them push with your thumb toward the ball of the foot. Do this several times. Do not let up pressure completely.

SECTION 13 TECHNIQUES
THE LIVER REFLEX= L

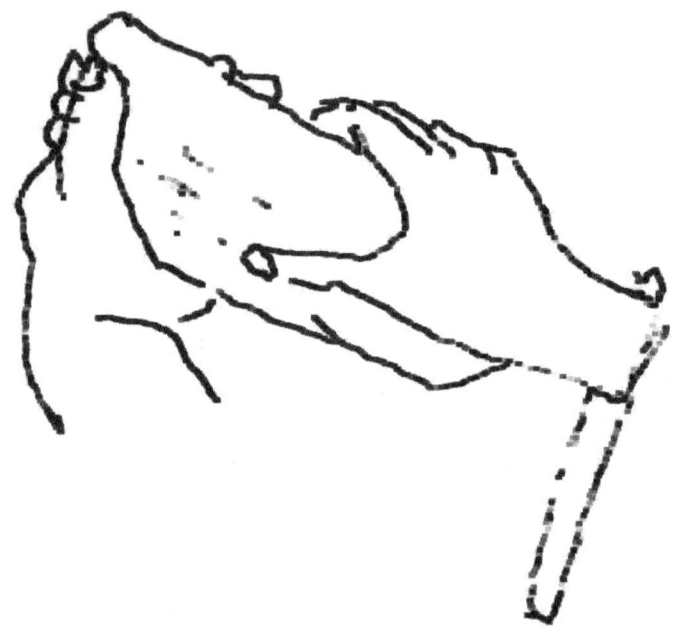

Since the liver is such a large organ the reflex area on the right foot is also large. Work the area slowly and deliberately. Be careful not to cause any real pain. The liver reflex area is only on the right sole. It is just below the ball of the foot and extends down to about ½ way between the base of the toes and the heel pad, from the inner edge down from the crease. Between the third and fourth toes and the area over the outer edge of the foot to the little toe. Use your thumb in a firm rolling pressure to cover the entire area. (This is an extremely large area). It is good to work both feet.

SECTION 14 TECHNIQUES
THE LUNG REFLEX= LU

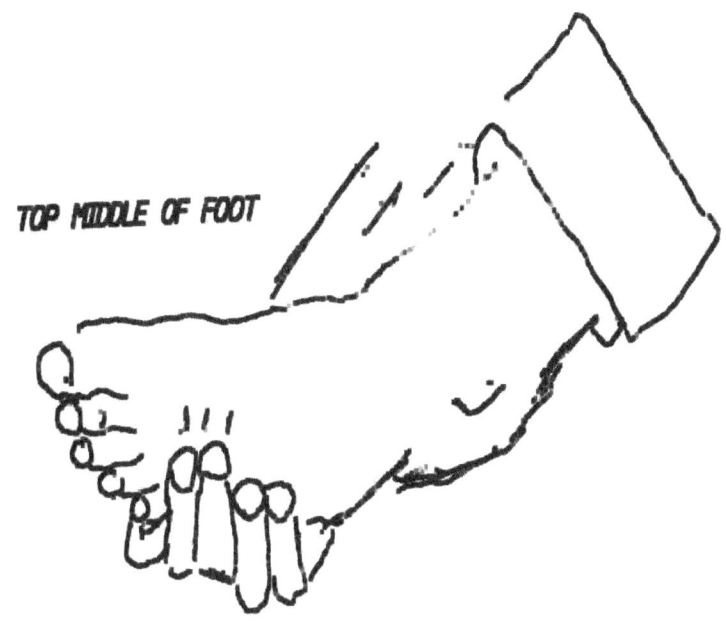

TOP MIDDLE OF FOOT

The lungs also cover a large area of the foot. Because there are two lungs it is good to work on both feet. The right foot affects the right lung. The left foot affects the left lung. The lung reflex is located on the soles of the feet at the base of the $2^{nd,}$ 3rd and 4th toes, and the groves between the pads. Start on the area under the second toe. Use your thumbs in a rolling motion as you press. (Control your breathing). Cover the entire area. The lung area is also on the top of the foot just above the base of the 2nd ,3rd and 4th toes. To work this area put the palm against the sole for resistance and use your middle and index fingers. Follow a press and release pattern. Gently press on top of the foot between the tendons of the toes. Do not use heavy pressure. This is also a large area so take your time and practice.

SECTION 15 TECHNIQUES
THE LYMPATHATIC SYSTEM REFLEX= LS

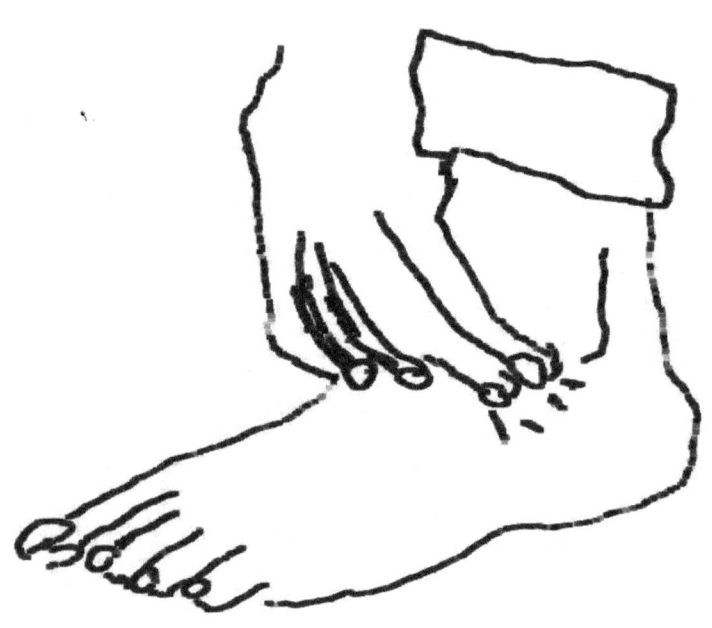

Since the lymphatic system plays such an important part in the immune system work this area well. The kidney and liver are very important. The reflex area for the lymphatic system can be found where the foot meets the ankle. The area extends from the inner ankle bone to the outer ankle bone. Start with your thumb on the inner ankle bone then use your finger tips on the outer ankle bone. Press in a circular motion gently as you move around the area. Note: You can gently roll the ankle in a circular motion. Be sure to cover the entire area gently. Take your time and practice.

SECTION 16 TECHNIQUES
OVARIES-TESTICLES= OT

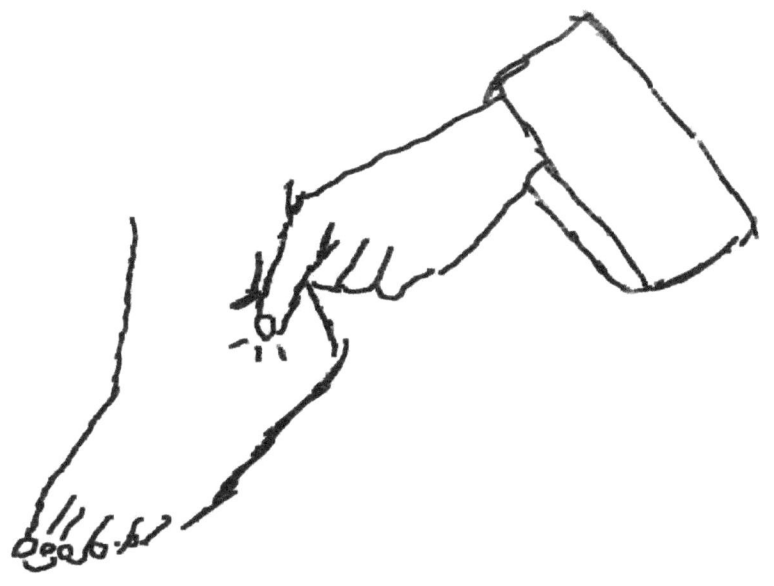

The reflex point for the ovaries and testicles are in the same place on the feet for both males and females. The point for the female are the ovaries, and the point for the male are the Testicles. The reflex point is located on both feet so it is good to work both feet. Work the hollows under the outer ankle bones just about the middle of each hollow. These are extremely sensitive areas so be careful when working on them. Place your thumb on the hollow under the inside ankle bone for resistance. Gently use your index finger and press firmly on the point, causing no pain of your own. Take your time and practice.

SECTION 17 TECHNIQUES
THE PANCREAS REFLEX= PA

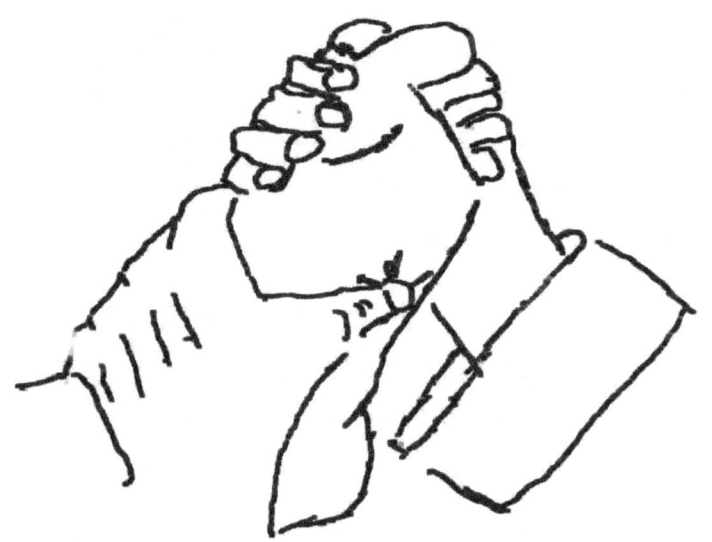

Although the pancreas is one gland it is located more or less in the center of the body. This means that the points are on both feet. The reflex area on the left foot is larger than the reflex point on the right foot. Be sure to work the entire organ in a session. Exert a firm pressure and be careful not to cause any pain from your pressure. This area is usually extremely sore when it has not been worked. The pancreas point reflex on the right sole is in the arch of the foot, about halfway between the base of the toes and the heel. It extends from the crease between the big and 2nd toe, to the inside edge of the foot. On the left foot it is in the same location but extends from the 4th toe over to the inside edge of the foot. Use your hand to gently hold the toes and push towards the ball of the foot with your thumb using a firm rolling pressure. Cover the entire area from the toes to the outer edge of the foot. Press slowly and gently. Do not release the pressure completely until you have finished.

SECTION 18 TECHNIQUES
THE PITUITARY REFLEX= PG

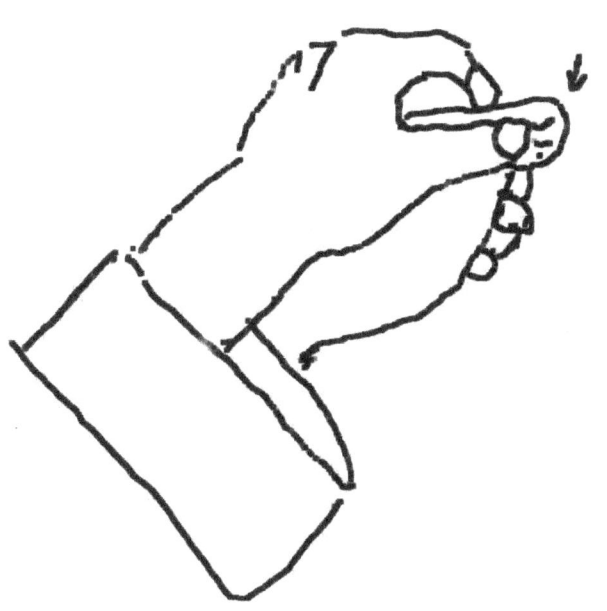

The pituitary reflexes are small specific points about the size of a sesame seed. It is difficult to stimulate them without working the other points. However this is actually quite good for you to work them all. Work the reflex points on both feet. The pituitary is located in the center of the skull and the point is split into (2) sides. The pituitary points are found in the center of the pads of the big toe, Grip the toe between your thumb and index finger. Use your thumb to press firmly against the point. Be sure to work both feet.

SECTION 19 TECHNIQUES
THE SINUS REFLEX= SIN

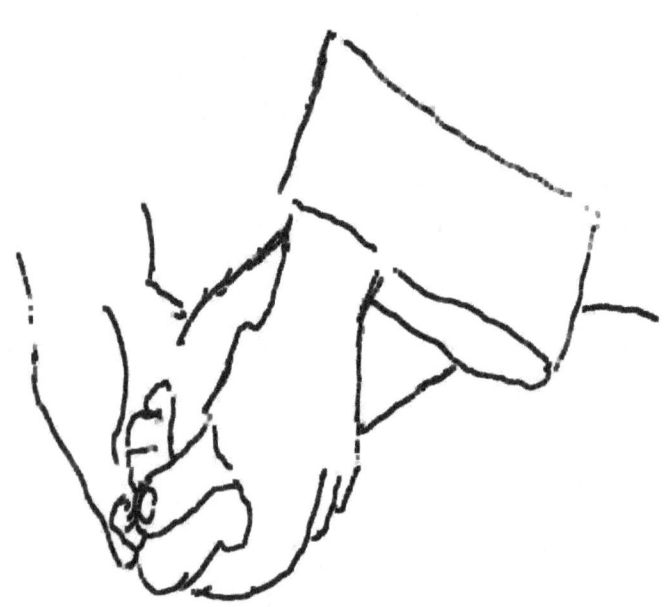

The sinus reflex is very beneficial. Take your time and work all the sinus areas. The sinus reflex areas are on both feet. Sinus are the top knuckles of the end of the toe. Work the pads, tips and side nails of the toe. For support first place the index and middle fingers of one hand on the nail of the toe to be worked. This gives enough support, then press gently but firmly. Do not cause pain as this is very tender. Take your time and practice. Be sure to work all the toes because you will also be working other reflexes that are beneficial. Keep a firm but gently pressure until soreness is relieved. This may take several treatments.

SECTION 20 TECHNIQUES
THE SCIATIC REFLEX= SN

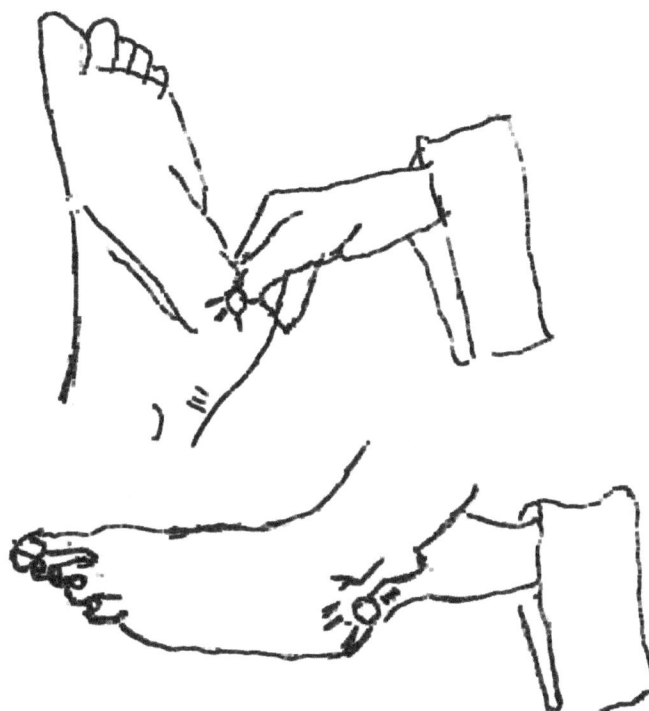

The sciatic nerves are very important, rather than work just one side when you have a problem always work both sides. The sciatic points are in three places on the feet.

1. The strips running underneath and behind the outer and inner ankle bones.
2. The narrow bands in the middle of the heel-pads that extend across the heel from edge to edge.
3. On the heel pad use the tip of your thumb firmly on the heel and grasp the heel in one hand. Use your index and middle fingers on the base of the heel. Use your thumb on the strip of the heel across from edge to edge just above the heel-pad. Work the base and area above the pad. Gently press harder on the heel but use a firm pressure. Do not cause pain.

SECTION 21 TECHNIQUES
THE SOLAR PLEXUX-DIAPHRAGM REFLEX= SP

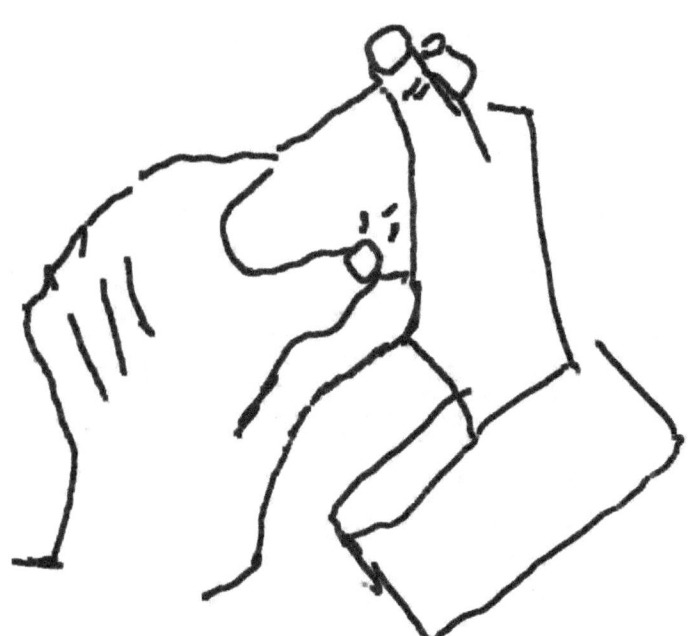

This is a good reflex area to work for stress and relaxation. The solar plexus also enhances a slow rhythmic breathing when worked slowly and gently. This area should be worked on with every treatment of the feet. The reflex points for the diaphragm and solar plexus are on both feet located in the center just below the balls of the feet. Place your thumb firmly on the reflex and use your other hand to flex the toes. Use your entire hand and wrist to press and rotate the thumb. Do this slowly and use firm pressure..

SECTION 22 TECHNIQUES
THE SPINE REFLEX= S

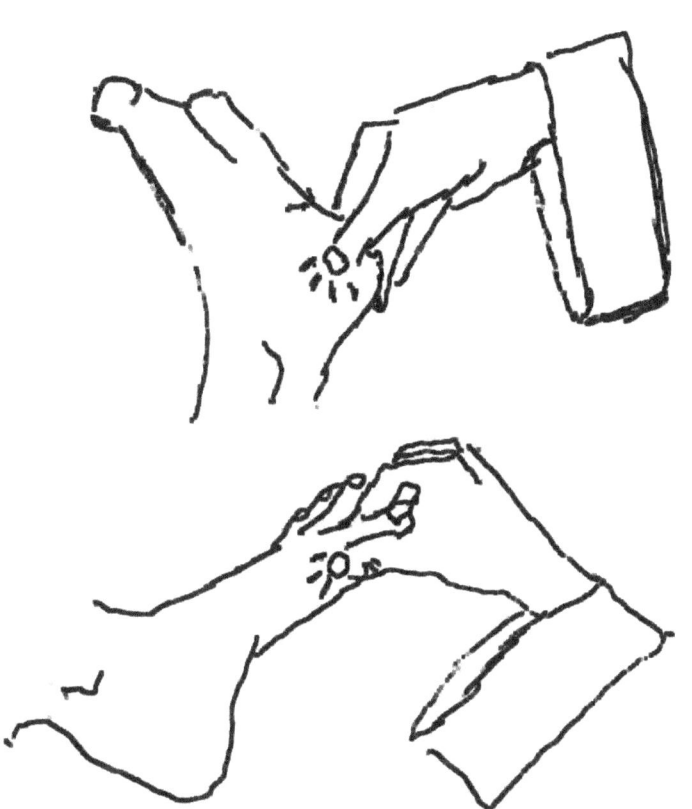

The spine and spinal cord are located on the midline of the body the reflex points are in both the right and left foot. The spine reflexes are along the inner edges of the feet and from the middle of the big toenails down to the bottom edges of the heels. Work the entire area with your thumb using a firm pressure. Start at the edge of the toenail and work down to the bottom of the heel in one pass.

SECTION 23 TECHNIQUE
THE SPLEEN REFLEX= SPL

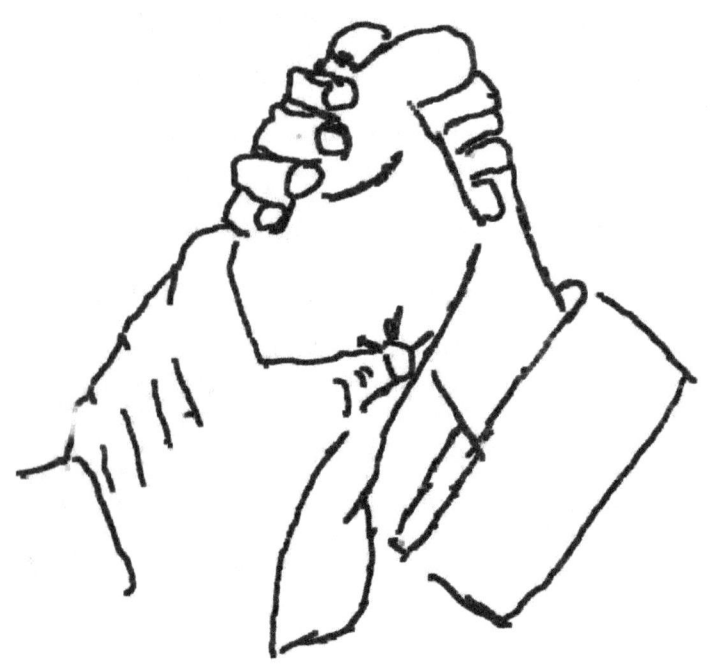

Because the spleen is found on the left side of the body the reflex point is on the left side only. However it is good to work both sides. The spleen reflex point that is on the left foot is just about ½ way between the base of the toes and the back of the heel. It extends from the crease between the 3rd and 4th toes over to the edge of the foot, just under the little toe. Use one hand to hold all the toes and push gently toward the ball of the foot. Press on the reflex area with the thumb of your other hand and use a firm pressure. Do not completely release pressure until finished. Put a little bend in the toes only as support.

SECTION 24 TECHNIQUE
THE STOMACH REFLEX= STO

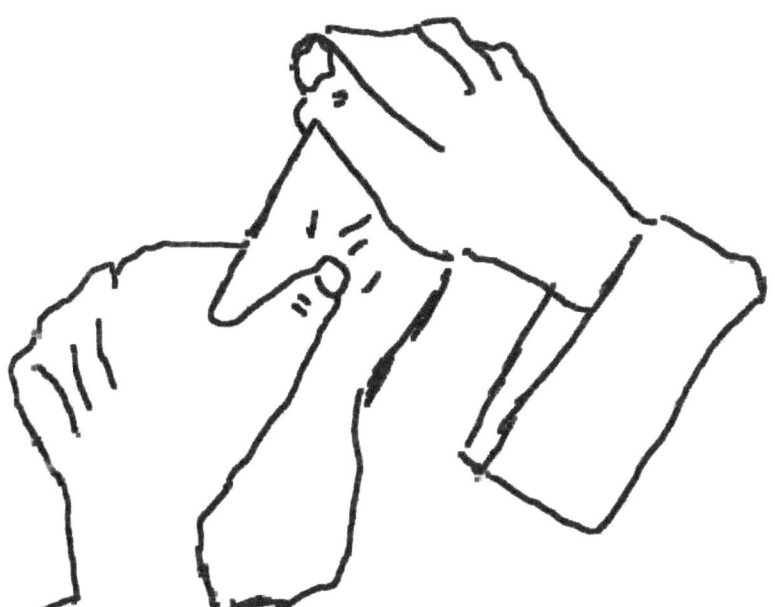

The stomach reflex on the left foot is a broad area. While on the right it is much smaller. This corresponds to the para portions of the stomach on the left and right sides. To find the stomach points on the left and right foot, divide the sole into quarters between the toes and heel. The reflex area is in the second quarter down from the toes below the ball of the foot and it extends from the edge under the big toe over to directly below the crease between the 3rd and 4th toe. (Note it is advised to use both thumbs and support the foot with your fingers). There is an illustration of the chart of quartering in the back of this manual. Use a firm thumb pressure.

SECTION 25 TECHNIQUES
THE THYROID-PARATHYROID REFLEX= PTG

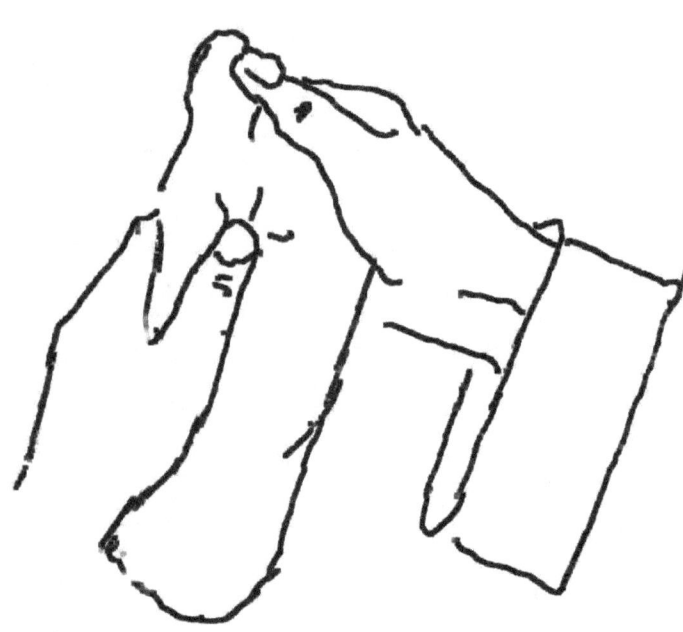

Both the thyroid and parathyroid glands are located along the body's mid-line section, with lobes on each side of the neck. The reflex points are on both feet. Be sure to work both right and left sides. The thyroid and parathyroid glands reflex points are found at the lower inside edge of the pad at the base of the big toe, straight down from the crease and between the big toe and 2nd toe. Be sure to use a gentle but firm thumb pressure. Be careful not to bruise any tissues or you might find yourself limping. Use your thumb in a pressing motion starting with only a little pressure and gently increasing it as you go.

.

SECTION 26 TECHNIQUES
THE UTERUS-PROSTATE REFLEX= UP

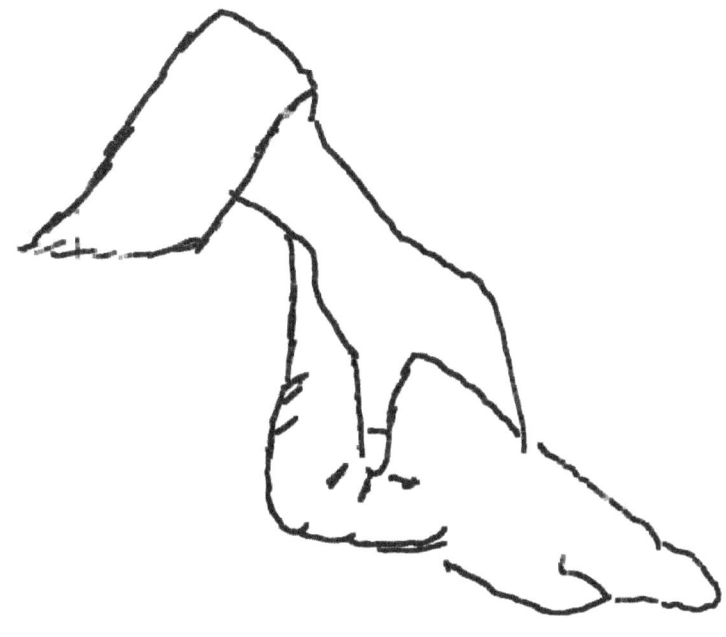

The points for the uterus and prostate are in the same places on both feet. The uterus and prostate points on both feet are in the hollows under the inner ankle bones just about the middle of each hollow. These are extremely sensitive areas. Be sure to work both the left and the right sides of the foot in a session. Place your thumb on the hollow under the inside ankle bone. Press gently but firmly on the reflex. Practice very carefully while holding the foot in the other hand for support.

DEFINITIONS

1. AG= ADRENL GLANDS
2. AS= ARMS SHOULDERS
3. BUU= BLADDER- URETHERS-URETHRA
4. B= BRAIN
5. BR= BREASTS
6. E= EARS
7. EY= EYES
8. GB= GALLBLADDER
9. H= HEART
10. HTL= HIPS-THIGHS- LEGS
11. IN= INTESTINE
12. K= KIDNEY
13. L= LIVER
14. LU= LUNGS
15. LS= LYMPHATIC SYSTEM
16. OT= OVARIES- TESTICLES
17. PA= PANCREAS
18. PG= PITUITARY GLAND
19. SIN= SINUSES
20. SN= SCIATIC NERVES
21. SP= SOLAR PLEXUS
22. S= SPINE
23. SPL= SPLEEN
24. STO=STOMACH
25. PTG= THYROID-PARATHYROID GLANDS
26. UP= UTERUS-PROSTATE

CHART 1

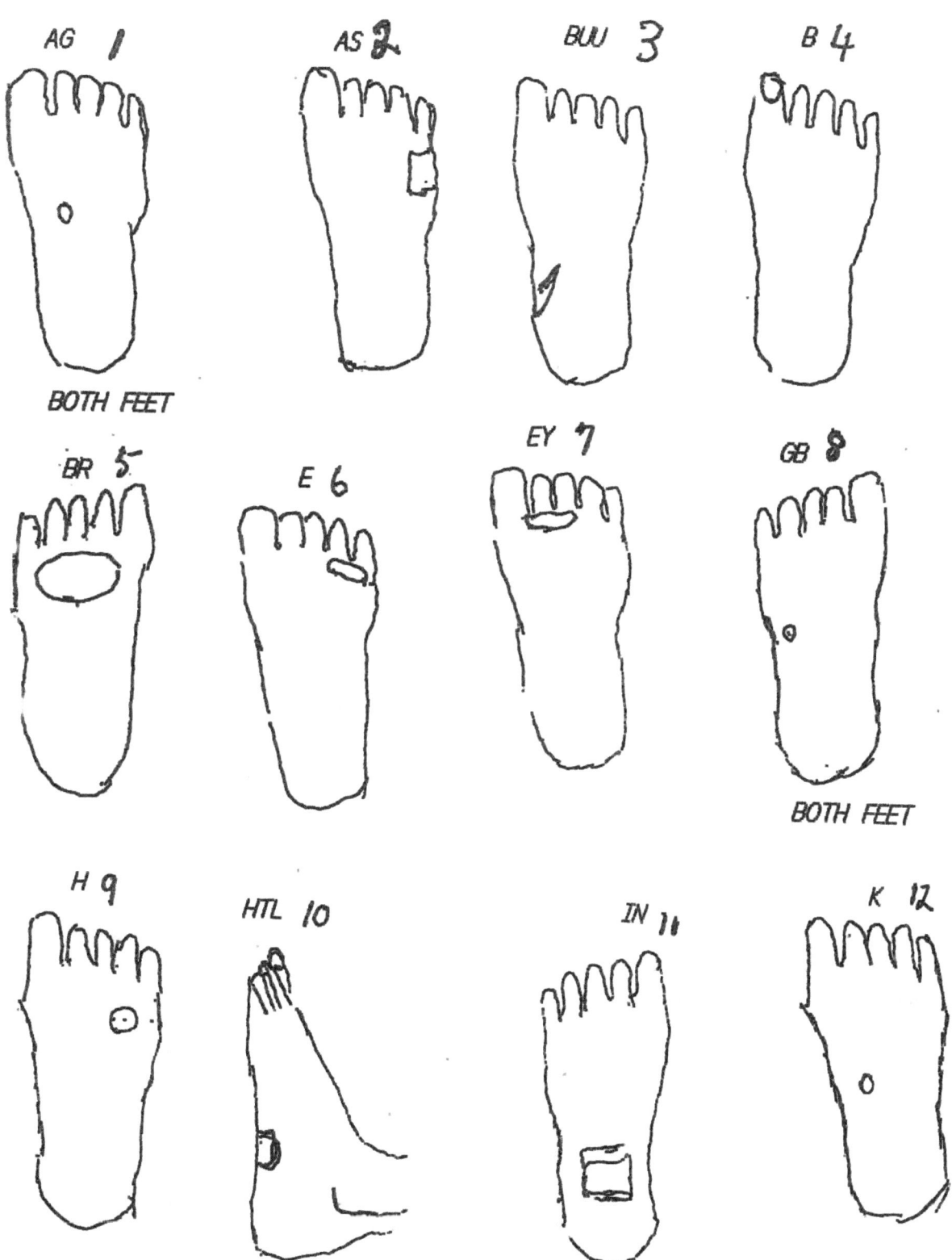

CHART 2

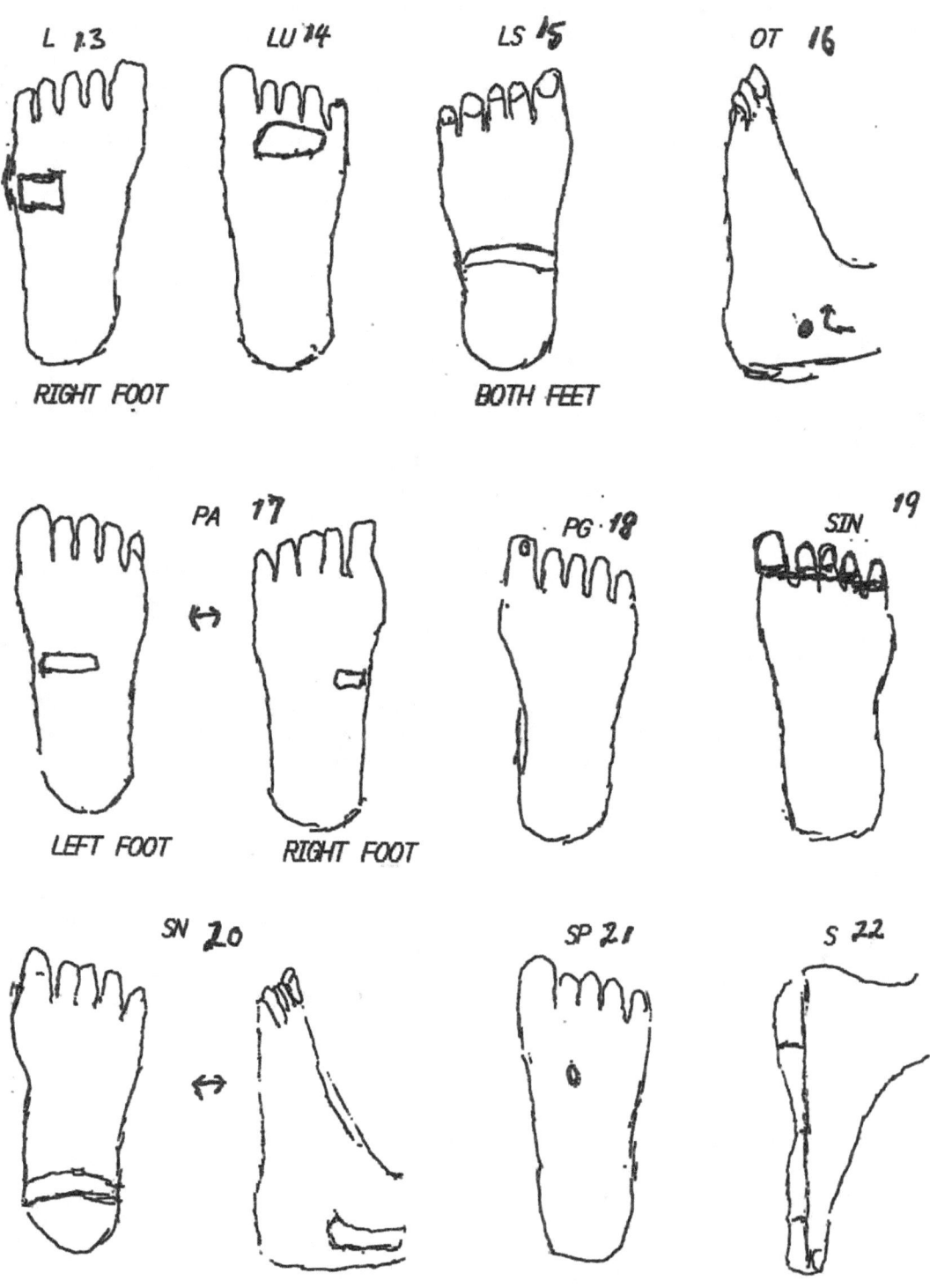

CHART 3

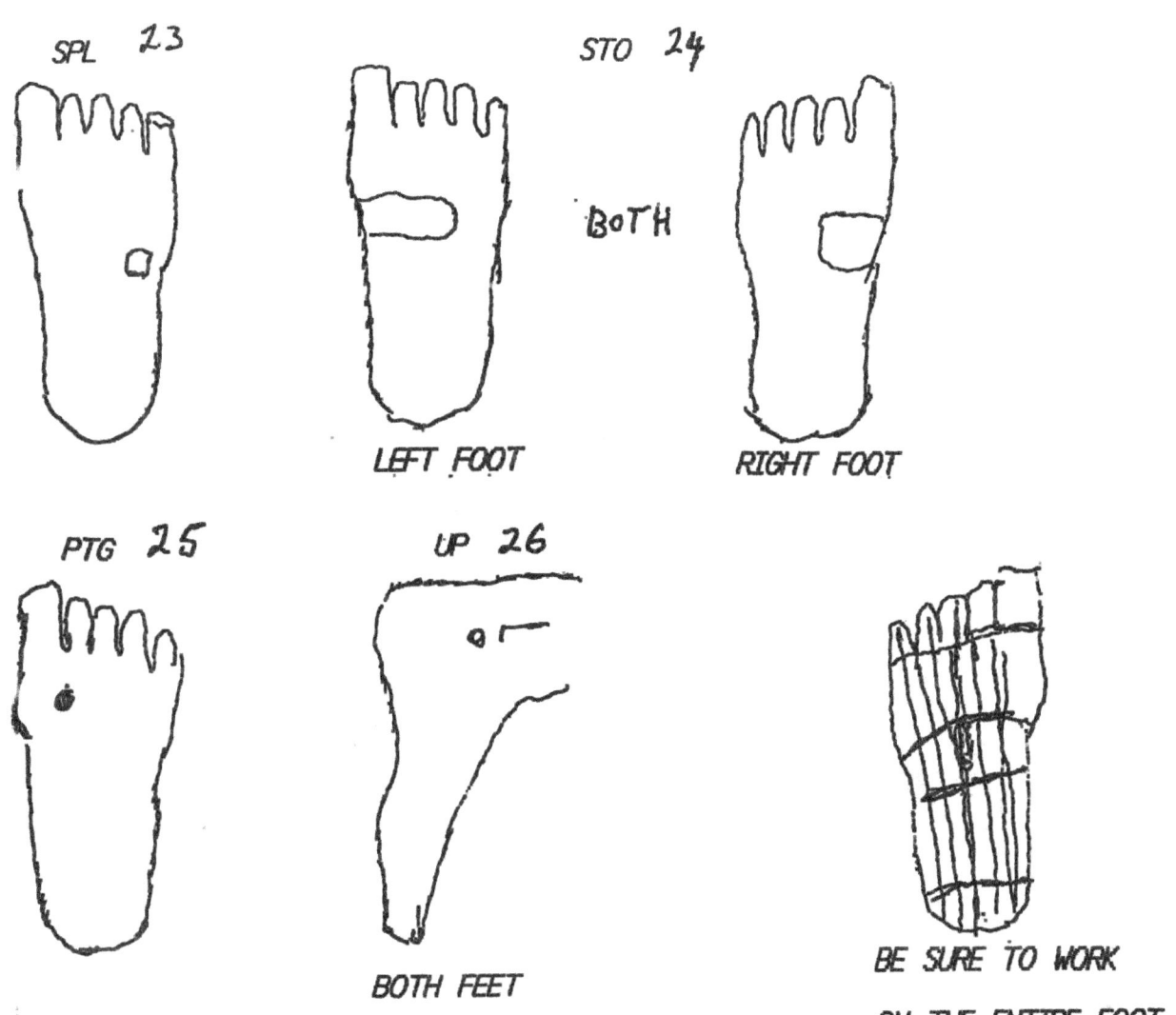

SPL 23

STO 24

BOTH

LEFT FOOT

RIGHT FOOT

PTG 25

UP 26

BOTH FEET

BE SURE TO WORK
ON THE ENTIRE FOOT.

SHIATSU TOM & REIKI MARIE HEALING ARTS SCHOOLS DIRECTORY
WE ARE NOT AFFILIATED WITH ANY OF THE SCHOOLS. THE PURPOSE OF THIS DIRECTORY IS TO OFFER HELPFUL INFORMATION.

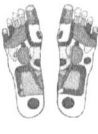

IN HEALTH
1309 HILLCREST DR
ANCHORAGE, AK 99503

CONTACT: KATHY UNGERECHT
PHONE: 907-278-4646
E-MAIL: KATHY@INHEALTHALASKA.COM
WEBSITE: HTTP://WWW.INHEALTHALASKA.COM

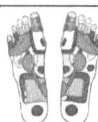

AMERICAN ACADEMY OF REFLEXOLOGY
13315 W WASHINGTON BOULEVARD
LOS ANGELES, CA

CONTACT: BILL FLOCCO
PHONE: (818) 841-7741
E-MAIL: REFLEXOLOGYEDU@AOL.COM
WEBSITE: HTTP://AMERICANACADEMYOFREFLEXOLOGY.COM

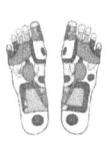

MODERN INSTITUTE OF REFLEXOLOGY
4086 YOUNGFIELD
WHEAT RIDGE, CO 80033

CONTACT: ZACHARY BRINKERHOFF
PHONE: 1-800-533-1837
E-MAIL: ZACHARY@REFLEXOLOGYINSTITUTE.COM
WEBSITE: HTTP://WWW.REFLEXOLOGYINSTITUTE.COM

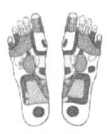

JUST FOR HEALTH SCHOOL OF REFLEXOLOGY AND HEALING ARTS
3502 S. CORONA ST #1
ENGLEWOOD, CO 80113

CONTACT: RACHEL LORD

PHONE: 303-320-4367
E-MAIL: JUSTFORHEALTH7@GMAIL.COM
WEBSITE: HTTP://WWW.JUSTFORHEALTH.NET

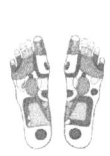

ACADEMY OF ANCIENT REFLEXOLOGY
4811 SERENA CIRCLE
SAINT. AUGUSTINE, FL 32084

CONTACT: KAREN BALL
PHONE: 904-553-4067
E-MAIL: KAREN@ACADEMYOFANCIENTREFLEXOLOGY.COM
WEBSITE:
HTTP://WWW.ACADEMYOFANCIENTREFLEXOLOGY.COM

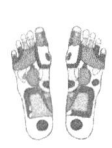

ACADEMY OF RADIANT HEALTH
6045 PATTINGHAM DRIVE
ROSWELL, GA 30075

CONTACT: KO TAN
PHONE: 770-843-2993
E-MAIL: KOTAN@ACADEMYOFRADIANTHEALTH.COM
WEBSITE: HTTP://WWW.ACADEMYOFRADIANTHEALTH.COM

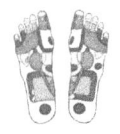

HEALTHY SOLES
2020 HILLSDOWN RD
DAVIS, IL 61019

CONTACT: SUSAN WATSON
PHONE: 866-737-2674
E-MAIL: HEALTHYSOLES@MCHSI.COM
WEBSITE: HTTP://WWW.HEALTHYSOLESSCHOOL.COM

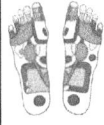

LAURA NORMAN
REFLEXOLOGY
FLORIDA,
MASSACHUSETTS AND NEW

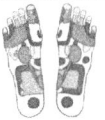

REFLEXOLOGY-PLUS
1590 17TH AVE
MARION, IA 52302-2376

YORK
DELRAY BEACH, FL 33483

CONTACT: LAURA NORMAN
PHONE: 561-272-1220
E-
MAIL: INFO@LAURANORMAN.CO
M
WEBSITE:
HTTP://WWW.LAURANORMAN.COM

CONTACT: PAT BARRANCE
PHONE: 319-373-0345
E-
MAIL: PBARRANCE@JUNO.CO
M
WEBSITE: HTTP://REFLEXOLOGY-
PLUS.ORG

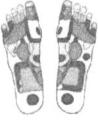

THE STONE INSTITUTE
2025 ZUMBEHL RD, PMB 20
ST. CHARLES, MO 63303

CONTACT: PAULA STONE
PHONE: 636-448-5579
E-
MAIL: STONEINSTITUTE@YAHOO.C
OM
WEBSITE:
HTTP://STONEINSTITUTE.REFLEXOL
OGY-USA.ORG/

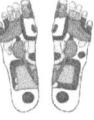

REFLEXOLOGY
CERTIFICATION
INSTITUTE
32945 DETROIT ROAD
AVON, OH 44011-2017

CONTACT: JOHN
HEIDENREICH
PHONE: (216) 299-1881
E-
MAIL: RCIJOHN924@GMAIL.
COM

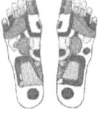

REFLEXOLOGY
SCIENCE
INSTITUTE
1170 OLD HENDERSON
RD, STE 206
COLUMBUS, OH 43220

CONTACT: BERIT
NILSSON
PHONE: 614-457-5783

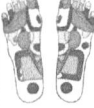

CAYCE/REILLY SCHOOL OF
MASSOTHERAPY
215-67TH ST
VIRGINIA BEACH, VA 23451

CONTACT: KAREN MEADE
PHONE: 757-428-3588 X7134
E-
MAIL: KAREN.MEADE@EDGARCAYCE.
ORG

E-MAIL: BERITNILS@AOL.COM	WEBSITE: HTTP://WWW.EDGARCAYCE.ORG/MASSAGESCHOOL/CE

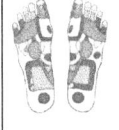

THE CENTER FOR UNIVERSAL REFLEXOLOGY
800 KNIBB ROAD
PASCOAG, RI 02859

CONTACT: THERESE MAGNAN
PHONE: 401-474-1457
MAIL: FOOTLADY99@VERIZON.NET
HTTP://REFLEXOLOGYSCHOOLRI.COM

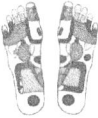

SEATTLE REFLEXOLOGY & MASSAGE CENTER
419 QUEEN ANNE AVE #107
SEATTLE, WA 98109

CONTACT: LISA HENSELL
PHONE: 206-297-6019
E-MAIL: LHENSELL@NETZERO.NET
WEBSITE: HTTP://WWW.SEATTLE-REFLEXOLOGY.COM

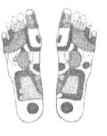

CRANIO SACRAL REFLEXOLOGY INTERNATIONAL
U.S. TEACHERS:DR. MARTINE FAURE-ALDERSON, MARILYN ALLING
EAST MOLESEY, KT8 OBU

CONTACT: TO SCHEDULE A CLASS IN YOUR STATE CONTACT: BRENDA MAKOWSKY
PHONE: 312-282-9648
E-MAIL: CSREFLEXOLOGY@YAHOO.CO
WEBSITE:
HTTP://CRANIOSACRALREFLEXOLOGYINTERNATIONAL.COM

THE REFLEXOLOGY MENTOR
CE DISTANCE TELECLASSES/WEBINARS
MANZANARES METHOD CLASSES,

CONTACT: LINDA CHOLLAR, AAED
PHONE: 310-318-3353
E-MAIL: LINDA@REFLEXOLOGYMENTOR.COM
WEBSITE:
HTTP://WWW.REFLEXOLOGYMENTOR.COM

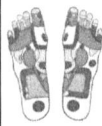

Alaska Reflexology Association

AKRA

1309 Hillcrest Dr
Anchorage, AK 99503
Contact Person: Kathy Ungerecht
Phone: 907-278-4646
Email: Kathy@inhealthalaska.com
Website: http://www.reflexology-usa.org/states/alaska.html

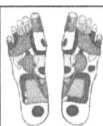

Arizona Reflexology Association

AZRA

7320 N. La Cholla Blvd, Ste 154, #145
Tucson, AZ 85741
Contact Person: Virginia Farwell
Phone: 520-722-1649
Email: info@reflexology-az.com
Website: http://www.reflexology-az.com

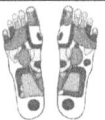

Reflexology Association of California

RAC

PO Box 4286

Lakewood, CA 90711
Contact Person: Rhonda Funes
Phone: 310-899-6289
Email: RACreflexology@yahoo.com
Website: http://www.reflexology-ca.org

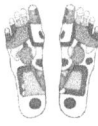 **Associated Reflexologists of Colorado**

ARC

PO Box 697
Englewood, CO 80151
Contact Person: Elizabeth An Heard
Phone: 303-745-0430
Email: Elizabeth@reflexology-colorado.org
Website: http://www.reflexology-colorado.org

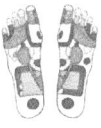 **Reflexology Association of Connecticut**

RACT

c/o 250 Wolcott Road
Wolcott, CT 06716
Contact Person: Joan Myers
Phone: 860-276-0517
Email: info@reflexologyct.org
Website:
http://www.reflexologyct.org

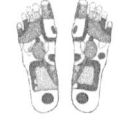 **Florida Association of Independent Reflexologists**

FAIR

PO Box 592
Hallandale Beach, FL 33008
Contact Person: Dayl Kumpa
Phone: 321-914-4169
Email: dp2730@gmail.com

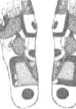 **Georgia Reflexology Organization**

GRO

P.O. Box 28031
Atlanta, GA 30358
Contact Person: Ko Tan
Phone: 770-843-2993
Email:
KoTan@AcademyofRadiantHealth.com
Website:
http://www.georgiareflexology.org/

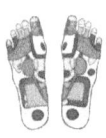

Reflexology Association of Hawaii

RAH
320 Liliuokalani Ave #802
Honolulu, HI 96815
Contact Person: Linda Friedman
Phone: 1-808-944-4588
Email: solecare88@yahoo.com

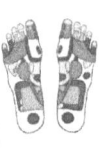

Parkersburg, IA 50665
Contact Person: Jamie L. Thompson
Phone: 319-830-4908
Email: toadilyjamie@aol.com

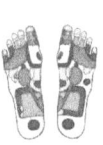

Reflexology Association of Illinois

RAI
Washington, IL 61571
Contact Person: Naomi Green, President
Phone: 309-648-2998
Email: reflexilrai@gmail.com
Website: http://www.reflexillinois.org

RAM
5009 Excelsior Blvd - Ste 101
St. Louis Park, MN 55416
Contact Person: Becket Olson
Email: hands2wk@yahoo.com
Website:
http://www.reflexologymn.com

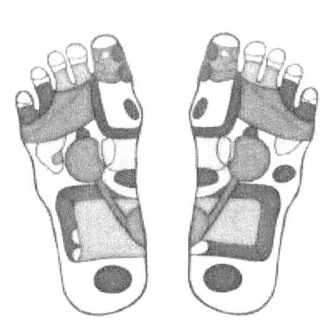

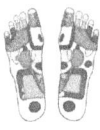 **North Carolina Reflexology Association**

NCRA
P.O. Box 25646
Charlotte, NC 28229-5646
Contact Person: Cyndi Hill
Phone: 704-636-4153
Email: cynthh152@aol.com
Website: http://www.reflexology-nc.org

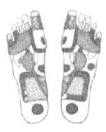 **North Dakota Reflexology Association**

NDRA
8661 156th Ave NE
Drayton, ND 58225
Contact Person: Jan Styles
Phone: 1-701-454-6495
Email: nd.reflexology@gmail.com
Website: http://www.reflexology-nd.com

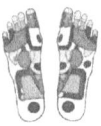 **New Mexico Association of Reflexologists**

NMAR
Santa Fe, NM 87505
Contact Person: Fred Coen
Phone: 505-982-4408
Email: fredcoen@cybermesa.com
Website:
http://web.mac.com/reflexon/NMAR

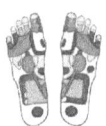 **New York State Reflexology Association**

NYSRA
, NY
Contact Person: Angelique Clarke
Phone: 646-805-8474
Fax: 516-2703531
Email: info@nysraweb.org
Website:
http://www.newyorkstatereflexology.org/

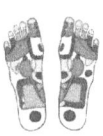 **Oregon Reflexology Network**

ORN
2556 East Side Rd.
Hood River, OR 97031
Contact Person: Marie Louise Penchoen
Phone: 541-386-7998
Email: info@ORNetwork.org
Website: http://www.oregonreflexologynetwork.org

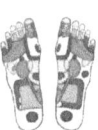 **Reflexology Association of Rhode Island**

RARI
Wakefield, RI 02879
Contact Person: Janine Deutsch
Phone: 401-829-8161
Email: janreflex@cox.net
Website: http://www.reflexologyri.com

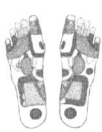 **Tennessee Reflexology Association**

TRA
11769 N. Williamsburg Drive
Knoxville, TN 37922
Contact Person: Ted Helms
Phone: 865-966-7989
Email: tch007@tds.net
Website: http://www.tnreflexology.org

WORKBOOK NOTES:

ABOUT THE AUTHORS:

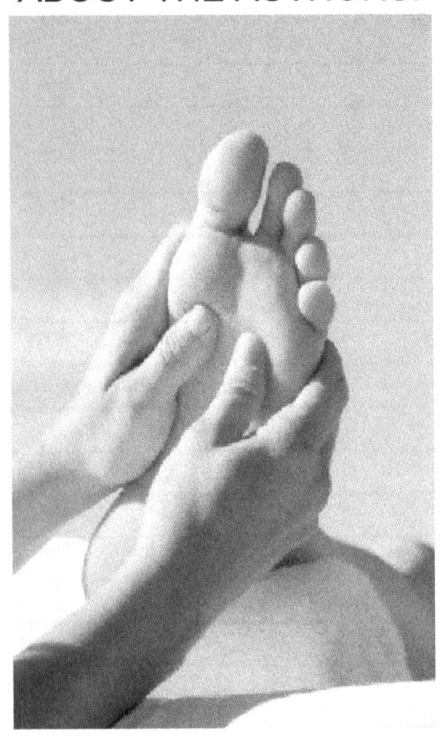

Both Shiatsu Tom and Reki Marie are both trained Physio-therapists with a background in the healing arts. Shiatsu Tom studied Shiatsu and acupuncture in Japan and started his training learning the art of reflexology. He also is a black belt in martial arts. He maintained a successful practice and office in San Bernardino, California for many years. He now teaches various modalities of the healing arts in Big Bear, CA and Sedona Arizona. He has been a practitioner of the healing arts with over 50 years of experience. Reiki Marie is a Reiki practitioner and instructor of the healing arts and she specializes in distant Reiki. She also has a background in Shaman healing practices. She has over 15 year of experience in the healing arts which includes Sports therapy, Reflexology and Shiatsu. Reiki Marie learned Shiatsu from Shiatsu Tom. She also studied acupuncture with Shiatsu Tom and had a successful healing practice for many years and now teaches.

Both Healing art practitioners reside in California but offer training for students of the healing arts in California and Sedona Arizona.

Email us or write to us for more information on how to obtain a certificate in Reflexology From Shiatsu Tom & Reiki Marie or information on other products or services.
Most course work is distant learning and some of our classes are taught in Big Bear, California or Sedona, Arizona.

Shiatsu (Tom)
P.O. Box 3279
Big Bear City, CA 92314

Email: shiatsutomreikimarie@gmail.com
Website: https://www.createspace.com/3863841

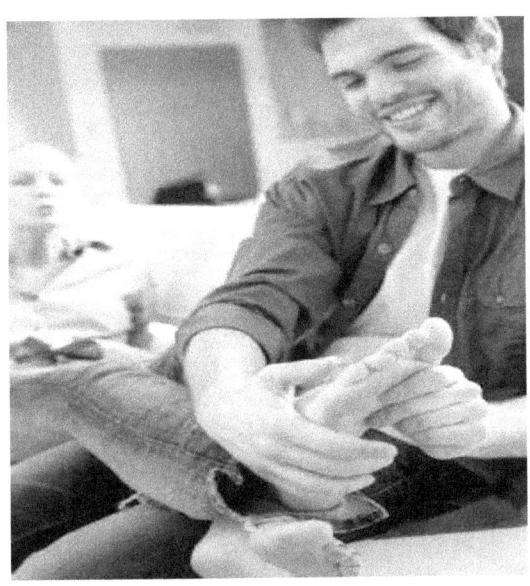

Copyright

BIBLIOGRAPHY
PHOTO ACKNOWLEDGEMENTS

FOOT MASSAGE

Wood stick massage by Satit Srihin

Inner Circle by Simon Howden

Man Massaging Womans Feet by Ambro

Foot by Simon Howden

Foot Massage by Markuso

Female Leg by photo stock

Opulent Background by Idea go

Massage photo by healingbdream

Reflexology Foot Massage by satit_srihin

Relaxing Foot On Bed by mack2happy

Reflexology history from Wikipedia, the free encyclopedia

The Devil's Kitchen sinkhole in Sedona, AZ photo By: SeanMD80-Wikipedia creative commons

Photo drawings illustration Shiatsu Tom & Reiki Marie